Table of Contents

1 Introduction to Gene Editing

Gene editing, a revolutionary approach to manipulating genetic material, holds immense potential for treating and preventing a myriad of diseases. This chapter will introduce the foundational technologies underpinning this powerful field, providing a comprehensive overview accessible to all. We will explore the mechanisms of several gene-editing systems, comparing and contrasting their strengths and weaknesses.

The development of gene editing technologies has accelerated rapidly in recent decades, moving from cumbersome methods to incredibly precise and efficient systems. Early techniques, such as zinc finger nucleases (ZFNs) and transcription activator-like effector nucleases (TALENs), involved creating custom proteins that could bind to specific DNA sequences and cut the DNA at a precise location. While these methods proved groundbreaking, designing and producing these proteins was a complex and time-consuming process, limiting their widespread adoption. The cost and complexity associated with their design and manufacture, coupled with lower efficiency compared to newer methods, significantly hampered their use. Moreover, the potential for off-target effects – unintended cuts at other locations in the genome – posed significant challenges. Despite their limitations, ZFNs and TALENs played a crucial role in paving the way for more advanced gene editing tools.

Then came CRISPR-Cas systems, a game-changer in the field. CRISPR, which stands for Clustered Regularly Interspaced Short Palindromic Repeats, is a naturally occurring bacterial defense mechanism adapted for gene editing. The system utilizes a guide RNA molecule, which is easily programmable to target specific DNA sequences, paired with the Cas9 protein, a molecular scissor that cuts the DNA at the targeted location. This simple yet elegant design offers several advantages over previous methods: it's significantly cheaper and faster to design and implement, it boasts higher editing efficiency, and it has demonstrated remarkable precision, significantly reducing off-target effects. However, even with CRISPR's considerable advancements, challenges remain. The potential for off-target edits, while reduced, still exists and requires careful monitoring and optimization. Furthermore, delivering the CRISPR-Cas system to the target cells or tissues in the body remains a significant hurdle, particularly for in vivo applications.

Understanding the intricacies of gene editing requires grasping the basic mechanisms of DNA repair. When the Cas9 protein cuts the DNA, the cell's natural repair mechanisms kick in. These mechanisms, primarily non-homologous end joining (NHEJ) and homology-directed repair (HDR), can be exploited for different purposes. NHEJ is an error-prone repair pathway that often introduces small insertions or deletions at the cut site, potentially disrupting the gene's function. This is a useful tool for gene knockout studies or gene disruption therapies. In contrast, HDR offers a more precise approach by utilizing a provided DNA template to repair the break, allowing for the precise insertion or replacement of genetic material. This targeted repair enables gene correction or gene addition, expanding the therapeutic potential significantly. Choosing the appropriate repair pathway and optimizing the editing process are critical factors determining the success of gene editing strategies.

The future of gene editing holds immense promise. Ongoing research focuses on improving targeting specificity, enhancing delivery methods, and exploring new applications. Scientists are actively developing novel Cas proteins with improved properties and expanding the range of target sequences accessible through CRISPR-Cas systems. Advancements in delivery methods, including the development of more efficient viral vectors and non-viral delivery systems, are crucial for translating gene editing technologies into effective therapies. The potential applications extend far beyond the treatment of genetic diseases, encompassing areas like cancer immunotherapy, agricultural biotechnology, and even basic biological research. However, realizing this potential requires careful consideration of the ethical and societal implications, rigorous safety testing, and the establishment of robust regulatory frameworks. Ultimately, the responsible and ethical development and application of gene editing technologies are paramount to ensuring its benefits are widely accessible while mitigating potential risks. The journey towards harnessing the full potential of gene editing is a complex one, but the advancements made so far demonstrate the immense promise this technology holds for reshaping the future of medicine and beyond.

1.1 CRISPR-Cas Systems

CRISPR-Cas systems, derived from bacterial defense mechanisms, represent a revolutionary gene-editing technology. Their simplicity and efficiency have propelled them to the forefront of genetic engineering, surpassing older methods like ZFNs and TALENs in both precision and ease of use. This ease of application stems from the programmable nature of the system; a guide RNA molecule directs the Cas enzyme, usually Cas9, to a specific DNA sequence, allowing for targeted modifications. Unlike earlier methods requiring extensive protein engineering for each target site, CRISPR-Cas simplifies the process significantly.

The mechanism involves the guide RNA forming a complex with the Cas enzyme, which then recognizes and binds to the complementary DNA sequence. Once bound, Cas9 creates a double-stranded break in the DNA. The cell's natural DNA repair mechanisms then kick in, either through non-homologous end joining (NHEJ), which is error-prone and often results in small insertions or deletions, or through homology-directed repair (HDR), which utilizes a provided DNA template for precise gene correction or insertion. This duality makes CRISPR-Cas versatile; NHEJ allows gene disruption, while HDR allows for precise edits.

However, this precision is not absolute. Off-target effects, where the CRISPR-Cas system edits unintended DNA sequences, remain a significant challenge. These off-target events can have unpredictable consequences, ranging from minor functional changes to potentially harmful mutations. Therefore, meticulous guide RNA design and optimization are critical to minimizing such risks. Researchers continuously develop improved guide RNA selection algorithms and Cas enzyme variants with enhanced specificity to mitigate this problem. Sophisticated computational tools and in vitro assays are employed to predict and assess potential off-target sites before in vivo applications.
Furthermore, the delivery of the CRISPR-Cas components to the target cells presents another hurdle. Viral vectors, while efficient, carry risks associated with immunogenicity and insertional mutagenesis. Non-viral methods such as lipid nanoparticles and electroporation offer safer alternatives, but their delivery efficiency is often lower, especially for in vivo applications targeting specific tissues or organs. The ongoing research and development in nanotechnology and targeted delivery systems aim to enhance the efficiency and safety of non-viral approaches. Combining advanced delivery systems with refined CRISPR-Cas systems is essential for advancing clinical applications.
The therapeutic potential of CRISPR-Cas systems is vast. In oncology, it shows promise in developing targeted cancer therapies, enhancing immune cell function to attack tumor cells, and even correcting genetic defects driving cancer development. Hematological disorders, like sickle cell anemia and beta-thalassemia, have seen remarkable advancements, with CRISPR-based ther-

apies demonstrating significant clinical success. Moreover, inherited metabolic disorders and monogenic diseases, often characterized by single gene defects, represent promising targets for CRISPR-mediated gene correction. The successful treatment of these conditions holds the potential to profoundly impact individuals' lives.

Despite its immense potential, ethical considerations warrant careful attention. Germline editing, modifying the genes in reproductive cells that are passed down to future generations, raises profound ethical concerns about unintended consequences and the potential for altering the human gene pool. The debate surrounding germline editing is ongoing, necessitating robust regulatory frameworks to guide research and clinical applications responsibly. A global consensus on ethical guidelines and strict regulations is essential to ensure that the benefits of this technology are realized while avoiding potential harms. Public engagement and open discussions are paramount in shaping the responsible future of gene editing technologies.

In conclusion, CRISPR-Cas systems represent a powerful tool with the potential to transform medicine and various scientific fields. However, the challenges associated with off-target effects, delivery systems, and ethical considerations necessitate a cautious and responsible approach. Ongoing research focused on improving specificity, developing more efficient delivery methods, and establishing robust regulatory frameworks will be critical in realizing the full therapeutic potential of this revolutionary technology while addressing its associated complexities. The future of gene editing hinges on balancing the pursuit of scientific advancements with the ethical considerations inherent in manipulating the very building blocks of life. The ultimate goal is to harness this power for the benefit of humanity, ensuring equitable access and minimizing potential risks. A collaborative effort between scientists, ethicists, policymakers, and the public is vital to navigate these challenges and responsibly shape the future of gene editing.

1.2 ZFNs and TALENs

Zinc finger nucleases (ZFNs) and transcription activator-like effector nucleases (TALENs) represent earlier gene-editing technologies, paving the way for the more widely adopted CRISPR-Cas systems. Understanding their mechanisms and limitations offers valuable insight into the evolution of gene editing and highlights the challenges overcome in achieving precise genome modification. While less prevalent now, their historical significance remains crucial for a complete understanding of the field. These systems rely on engineered nucleases, proteins capable of cutting DNA at specific sequences. ZFNs utilize zinc finger proteins, small domains that bind to specific DNA triplets. Multiple zinc fingers are linked together to create a larger protein that recognizes a longer, unique DNA sequence. This targeted protein is fused to the FokI restriction enzyme, a nuclease that cuts DNA only when present as a dimer. Therefore, two ZFNs are necessary—one targeting each strand of the DNA double helix near the desired modification site. The FokI dimers create a double-strand break (DSB), stimulating the cell's natural DNA repair mechanisms, either non-homologous end joining (NHEJ), which often introduces insertions or deletions (indels) leading to gene disruption, or homology-directed repair (HDR), which allows for precise gene correction using a supplied DNA template. This careful design allows for accurate targeting, but creating effective ZFNs demands considerable expertise and can be costly and time-consuming.

TALENs, on the other hand, leverage transcription activator-like effector (TALE) proteins from plant pathogens. These proteins feature a modular architecture, with each repeat unit specifically recognizing a single DNA base. This modularity allows for easier design and construction of TALENs targeting longer sequences compared to ZFNs, offering increased specificity. Similar to ZFNs, a pair of TALENs is required to create a DSB, utilizing the FokI nuclease for cleavage. However, the modular design simplifies the process of constructing TALENs and offers more flexibility in targeting diverse DNA sequences.

Despite their advantages, ZFNs and TALENs present inherent limitations. Both systems can suffer from off-target effects, where the nucleases unintentionally cut DNA at unintended sites within the genome, potentially leading to undesirable mutations. The design process for both ZFNs and TALENs, although improved with TALENs, is still relatively complex and expensive compared to the simplicity of CRISPR-Cas systems. Their efficiency can also be variable, depending on the target sequence and cellular context, leading to inconsistent gene editing outcomes. This lack of widespread standardization hindered broader application compared to CRISPR, which offers greater ease of use and reduced overall costs, enabling wider access and applications across various research and clinical settings.

In the realm of clinical applications, ZFNs and TALENs have seen limited use, mainly due to the rise of CRISPR. While early attempts explored therapeutic interventions, their complexities hindered widespread translation. Despite showing early promise in specific gene correction contexts, their cumbersome design and off-target effects have made them less attractive compared to the more readily available and efficient CRISPR technology. However, the foundational knowledge and techniques developed through ZFN and TALEN research significantly contribute to our current understanding of gene editing and have laid the groundwork for the technological advancements witnessed in recent years. Understanding these earlier methods helps appreciate the significant leap forward that CRISPR-Cas represents, emphasizing the ongoing evolution and improvement in gene editing tools. Ultimately, the knowledge gained from these precursor technologies is indispensable to continue making progress in the field, refining techniques and ensuring that they are both safe and effective.

2 Personalized Medicine & Gene Editing

The convergence of gene editing and personalized medicine represents a paradigm shift in healthcare. No longer are treatments a one-size-fits-all approach; instead, we're moving towards therapies tailored to an individual's unique genetic makeup. This precision offers unprecedented opportunities to combat diseases previously considered incurable. Imagine a future where cancer is treated not with broad-spectrum chemotherapy, but with highly specific gene edits targeting only cancerous cells, minimizing harmful side effects. This isn't science fiction; it's the promise of personalized medicine powered by gene editing.

This individualized approach extends beyond cancer. Inherited genetic diseases, once a life sentence for affected individuals and their families, are becoming targets for gene correction therapies. Imagine preventing cystic fibrosis before symptoms even appear, or correcting the faulty gene responsible for Huntington's disease, halting its devastating progression. Gene editing offers the potential to eliminate these conditions entirely from family lines, rewriting the script of inherited illness. This represents hope for families facing generational burdens of disease. Pharmacogenomics, a field inextricably linked to gene editing, takes personalized medicine to another level. This area studies how an individual's genes affect their response to drugs. By analyzing a person's genetic code, doctors can predict which medications will be most effective and least likely to cause adverse reactions. Gene editing itself could play a role in engineering cells to enhance drug efficacy or reduce toxicity, opening avenues for creating safer and more powerful therapeutics. The future is less about a "one-size-fits-all" approach to prescriptions and more about tailored therapies created for each patient.

However, the path forward isn't without hurdles. The complexity of the human genome demands careful consideration of potential off-target effects–unintended changes to the genome that could have harmful consequences. Rigorous research, stringent safety protocols, and advanced gene editing technologies are crucial to minimizing these risks. Furthermore, equitable access to these life-changing therapies is paramount. The potential benefits of personalized medicine should be available to everyone, regardless of socioeconomic status or geographic location. We cannot allow a technological advancement to only benefit certain populations.

Ethical considerations are also critical. The ability to edit the human germline–the genes passed down to future generations–raises profound ethical questions. Societal discussions about the responsible use of these technologies are essential, ensuring ethical frameworks guide innovation and prevent misuse. We must establish clear guidelines to avoid inadvertently creating unintended consequences in the genetic makeup of future generations.

The integration of gene editing into clinical practice requires careful planning and execution. Clinical trials must be meticulously designed, with rigorous monitoring of patient safety and efficacy. Regulatory bodies must work collaboratively with researchers to ensure that therapies meet the highest safety standards before widespread implementation. Ultimately, the success of personalized medicine through gene editing hinges on a commitment to both scientific excellence and responsible innovation. It is a delicate dance between scientific advancement and ethical responsibility that will require collaborative efforts from researchers, regulators, and healthcare professionals. Ultimately, the collaborative focus will guide our path to ensuring both responsible research and effective deployment of these powerful technologies. The goal is to translate hope into tangible realities that change lives.

2.1 Cancer Treatment Advances

The landscape of cancer treatment is undergoing a dramatic transformation, largely fueled by advancements in gene editing technologies. No longer are we limited to broad-spectrum chemotherapies with their debilitating side effects; instead, we're moving towards highly targeted therapies tailored to an individual's unique genetic makeup. This personalized approach, enabled by precise gene editing tools like CRISPR-Cas9, allows us to directly address the genetic abnormalities driving cancerous growth.

Imagine a future where we can effectively silence oncogenes, those rogue genes fueling uncontrolled cell proliferation, or precisely repair tumor suppressor genes, the body's natural brakes against cancer development. This is no longer science fiction; it's the rapidly evolving reality of gene-edited cancer therapies. Researchers are exploring several avenues, including the development of CAR T-cell therapies, where a patient's own immune cells are genetically modified to specifically target and destroy cancer cells. The precision of gene editing drastically improves the effectiveness and reduces the risk of off-target effects compared to earlier approaches.

Furthermore, gene editing technologies offer a powerful tool in overcoming drug resistance, a significant challenge in cancer treatment. Cancer cells often develop mechanisms to evade the effects of chemotherapy or targeted therapies. Gene editing can help modify these resistance mechanisms, restoring the sensitivity of cancer cells to existing drugs or creating new therapeutic vulnerabilities. This opens up the possibility of repurposing existing drugs for improved efficacy or designing new drugs with enhanced effectiveness against specific cancer mutations.

However, the path to widespread clinical application is not without its hurdles. Delivering gene-editing tools to tumor cells effectively and safely remains a significant challenge. The immune system's response to the introduced genetic material is another crucial obstacle that needs further investigation and mitigation strategies. Off-target effects, although reduced with CRISPR compared to earlier technologies, still require rigorous monitoring and control to ensure patient safety.

One particularly promising area is the development of gene-edited vaccines. These vaccines are designed to trigger a strong and targeted immune response against specific cancer antigens, leading to the destruction of cancerous cells. Early clinical trials have shown encouraging results, demonstrating the potential of this approach to improve cancer treatment outcomes, even in advanced stages. The use of gene editing allows researchers to refine these vaccines, maximizing their efficacy and minimizing side effects.

The potential of gene editing in cancer treatment extends beyond direct targeting of cancer cells. It also holds promise in improving the efficacy of other cancer therapies, such as radiation therapy and immunotherapy. For instance, gene editing could enhance the sensitivity of cancer cells to radiation, allowing for lower doses and minimizing side effects. It can also be used to modify immune cells to improve their ability to recognize and destroy cancer cells. These approaches exemplify the versatile nature of gene editing technologies in revolutionizing oncology.

The integration of gene editing into routine cancer care requires a multifaceted approach. Robust preclinical studies are essential to assess the efficacy and safety of novel gene editing strategies. Furthermore, carefully designed clinical trials with rigorous monitoring are crucial for evaluating their effectiveness in diverse patient populations. Development of efficient and safe gene delivery systems must also continue apace, to overcome the significant biological barriers to widespread use.

The ethical considerations related to the use of gene editing in cancer treatment demand careful attention. Ensuring equitable access to these groundbreaking therapies is paramount, preventing the creation of a healthcare divide based on socioeconomic status or geographic location. Moreover, the potential for unintended long-term consequences necessitates rigorous monitoring and careful oversight. Ethical guidelines and regulatory frameworks must be constantly updated to keep pace with the rapid advancements in the field.

In conclusion, gene editing technologies represent a transformative paradigm shift in cancer treatment. While challenges remain, the potential benefits–highly targeted therapies, overcome drug resistance, and enhanced immunotherapies–are enormous. By addressing the current limitations and proceeding with caution and ethical consideration, we can harness the power of gene editing to significantly improve cancer treatment outcomes for patients worldwide, creating a future where cancer becomes a more manageable and even curable disease. The journey is complex, but the destination–a healthier future for countless individuals–is worth the continued effort. The convergence of genetic engineering, medical genetics, and biotechnology is ultimately bringing forth a revolution in healthcare, a revolution that is already impacting cancer care in profound and increasingly significant ways.

2.2 Genetic Disease Prevention

Genetic diseases, inherited flaws in our DNA, represent a significant challenge to human health. Understanding the mechanisms behind these diseases is crucial, and thankfully, advances in genetic engineering are providing new avenues for prevention. Early detection through carrier screening plays a vital role, allowing prospective parents to make informed decisions about family planning. This proactive approach minimizes the risk of passing on a deleterious gene.
For many couples, genetic counseling is invaluable. A genetic counselor can analyze family history, interpret test results, and discuss the implications of different genetic variants. This personalized guidance empowers couples to explore options such as preimplantation genetic diagnosis (PGD), where embryos created through in-vitro fertilization are screened for specific genetic defects. Only healthy embryos are then implanted, preventing the transmission of a disease.
Beyond PGD, pre-symptomatic testing, while offering a glimpse into one's future health, also poses challenges. Discovering a predisposition to a later-onset condition can lead to considerable psychological stress. Careful counseling and support networks are vital in such cases. For instance, an individual learning they have a high risk of developing Huntington's disease may need extensive psychological preparation to cope with the future implications, and this should be supported by a team of specialists.
The increasing accessibility of genetic testing necessitates a

heightened awareness among healthcare professionals. Doctors and nurses should be prepared to discuss the implications of genetic information with their patients, addressing anxieties and concerns. Furthermore, educational resources and training programs dedicated to the ethical and social aspects of genetic testing can help healthcare providers adequately support patients in understanding and utilizing these tests in a meaningful way. Open communication will foster trust and ensure appropriate patient choices.

Gene editing holds tremendous promise for preventing genetic diseases in the future. While still experimental, technologies like CRISPR-Cas9 offer the potential to directly correct genetic defects within an individual's genome. These interventions, however, remain complex and fraught with potential complications, like off-target effects and immune responses. Rigorous research and careful clinical trials are paramount to ensure the safety and efficacy of such procedures.

Currently, the focus lies on somatic gene editing – modifying genes in specific cells or tissues, without affecting germline cells and future generations. This approach reduces the ethical complexities of altering the human gene pool while still offering hope for treating a broad range of genetic disorders. Nevertheless, strict regulatory frameworks and ethical guidelines are needed to oversee research and clinical applications, ensuring responsible innovation and equitable access to these potentially life-changing technologies.

The field is rapidly evolving, and new discoveries are continually refining our understanding of genetic diseases and the potential for their prevention. Collaborative research involving genetic engineers, clinicians, ethicists, and policymakers is crucial to navigate the complex landscape of genetic disease prevention. Responsible innovation that benefits humanity requires a unified approach, ensuring the careful implementation of groundbreaking gene editing technologies. Constant advancements and refinements mean that staying informed on the developments is crucial.

For instance, researchers are actively exploring ways to improve the precision of gene editing tools, minimizing the risk of off-target edits and maximizing the therapeutic benefit. Simultaneously, efforts are underway to develop safer and more efficient gene delivery systems, ensuring the targeted modification of genes without causing unwanted side effects. These research priorities underscore the dynamic nature of the field and its continuous evolution.

In the long term, gene editing technologies could potentially transform the prevention and treatment of genetic diseases, fundamentally altering the trajectory of human health. However, the path forward requires careful consideration of ethical, societal, and regulatory implications. Open dialogue, transparency, and widespread collaboration will ensure the responsible development and implementation of this revolutionary technology. The potential benefits are immense; thus, addressing these complexities is essential.

Beyond technological advancements, addressing health disparities is crucial in ensuring that the benefits of gene editing technology are accessible to all populations regardless of their socioeconomic status or geographic location. Incorporating equity and inclusivity in the research, development, and clinical application phases is necessary to avoid widening existing health gaps, which is an important step towards fair implementation of this life-altering technology. This will lead to more ethical and equitable application.

2.3 Pharmacogenomics

Pharmacogenomics is revolutionizing how we approach drug development and treatment. It leverages our understanding of an individual's genetic makeup to predict their response to specific medications, paving the way for truly personalized medicine. This personalized approach minimizes adverse drug reactions, optimizes treatment efficacy, and ultimately improves patient outcomes. Instead of a one-size-fits-all approach, pharmacogenomics allows tailoring treatment to the unique genetic profile of each patient.

This powerful tool helps us understand why some individuals respond well to a drug while others experience severe side effects, or even no effect at all. These variations in drug response are often due to genetic differences affecting how the body processes medications– influencing drug metabolism, transport, and target interactions. By analyzing an individual's genes, we can identify potential variations that might predict a positive or negative response.

Consider a scenario involving warfarin, a common anticoagulant. Variations in genes encoding enzymes involved in warfarin metabolism can significantly influence the required dosage. Some individuals need a higher dose to achieve therapeutic efficacy while others are at risk of bleeding with standard doses. Pharmacogenomic testing can accurately determine the appropriate dose, improving safety and preventing complications. This is just one example of the many areas where pharmacogenomics significantly improves patient care.

The impact extends beyond dosage adjustments. Pharmacogenomics can also predict adverse drug reactions. Certain genetic variations can increase the risk of developing specific side effects from particular drugs. Knowing this in advance allows clinicians to proactively choose alternative medications, avoiding potential harm. Imagine the benefits of knowing a patient's genetic predisposition to a severe allergic reaction before prescribing a potentially problematic medication.

Beyond individual patient care, pharmacogenomics greatly influences drug development itself. Pharmaceutical companies are increasingly incorporating pharmacogenomic data into their research, identifying potential drug targets and designing drugs with improved safety and efficacy profiles. This approach helps companies avoid investing heavily in drugs that might fail due to unexpected adverse reactions in certain populations, a significant cost saver. The overall efficiency of the drug development process improves because drug discovery is guided by a deeper understanding of how genes influence drug response.

But implementing pharmacogenomics presents challenges. A major hurdle is the cost of genetic testing and the integration of pharmacogenomic data into clinical workflows. While the cost of genetic sequencing is steadily decreasing, the tests are still expensive enough to create barriers to widespread adoption. Clinicians also need training to interpret pharmacogenomic data and effectively integrate it into patient care. Furthermore, comprehensive databases correlating genetic variants with drug responses are necessary, and building and maintaining these is an extensive, ongoing effort.

Moreover, there are ethical considerations surrounding the storage, access, and interpretation of genetic data. Ensuring patient privacy and informed consent while also promoting open access to research data is a careful balancing act, necessitating stringent regulations and best practices. The potential for discrimination based on genetic information is also a concerning issue, and addressing this requires legislation and education to mitigate risks.

Despite these challenges, the future of pharmacogenomics is bright. As technology advances and costs decrease, genetic testing will become more accessible, and the integration of pharmacogenomics into routine clinical practice will become more seamless. The potential to improve patient safety, optimize treatment efficacy, and accelerate drug development is substantial. This personalized approach represents a major leap toward a future where healthcare is truly tailored to the individual, reflecting their unique genetic blueprint. The continuing development of sophisticated algorithms and bioinformatics tools will help clinicians and researchers interpret ever-growing amounts of genetic information. This will facilitate even more precise predictions of drug response, leading to better patient outcomes and a more efficient healthcare system.

3 Gene Therapy: Clinical Applications

Viral vectors, modified viruses stripped of their disease-causing capabilities, are currently the workhorses of gene therapy delivery. Their natural ability to infect cells and deliver genetic material makes them highly effective. Retroviruses, adeno-associated viruses (AAVs), and lentiviruses each present unique advantages and drawbacks. Retroviruses, for example, integrate their genetic payload into the host cell's DNA, ensuring long-term expression, but this integration can potentially disrupt existing genes. AAVs, on the other hand, offer less risk of insertional mutagenesis, but their carrying capacity for genetic material is limited. Lentiviruses, a subtype of retroviruses, provide a balance, capable of infecting both dividing and non-dividing cells, a crucial advantage for many target tissues. The choice of viral vector depends critically on the target cell type, the size of the therapeutic gene, and the desired duration of expression. Careful consideration of the vector's tropism–its ability to selectively infect certain cell types–is paramount for maximizing efficacy and minimizing off-target effects. Researchers are continually refining vector designs to enhance their targeting specificity and reduce potential adverse reactions. The field actively explores pseudotyping, modifying the viral surface proteins to alter their tropism and improve their ability to reach specific tissues.

Non-viral delivery methods offer an attractive alternative, bypassing some of the safety concerns associated with viral vectors. These methods, while generally less efficient than viral vectors, show promise and are actively being improved. Lipid nanoparticles (LNPs) encapsulate genetic material and are delivered to cells through endocytosis, the process by which cells engulf external particles. LNPs are particularly useful for delivering mRNA or small interfering RNAs (siRNAs), offering a temporary therapeutic effect. Electroporation, a physical method that uses brief electrical pulses to create temporary pores in cell membranes, allows the entry of therapeutic DNA or RNA. This method is relatively simple and versatile but often lacks the targeted delivery offered by viral vectors. Other non-viral methods include gene gun delivery, utilizing microscopic gold particles coated with DNA, and hydrodynamic injection, rapidly introducing large volumes of DNA solution into the bloodstream. The choice between viral and non-viral methods is a complex decision that must be made on a case-by-case basis, balancing the relative advantages and limitations of each approach in light of the specific therapeutic objective.

The successful application of gene therapy hinges significantly on the delivery system's ability to reach the target cells efficiently and safely. The delivery challenge varies dramatically depending on the disease and the target organ. For instance, delivering therapeutic genes to the brain poses unique difficulties due to the blood-brain barrier, a protective layer that restricts the entry of most substances. Similarly, targeting specific cell types within complex tissues like the liver or lungs presents significant challenges. Researchers are exploring various strategies to overcome these delivery hurdles, including the use of targeted ligands that enhance the specificity of viral vectors, the development of more efficient LNP formulations, and innovative methods for temporarily disrupting the blood-brain barrier. Furthermore, advancements in imaging techniques allow for real-time monitoring of vector delivery, assisting optimization and personalized dosing. This targeted delivery remains an active and critical area of research, with ongoing improvements aiming for more efficient and precise targeting strategies.

Beyond the choice of delivery vector, the development of effective gene therapy involves careful consideration of the therapeutic gene itself. The gene's sequence must be optimized for expression in the target cells, and its regulation must be carefully controlled to avoid unintended consequences. Promoters, sequences that control gene expression, are often engineered to restrict the expression of the therapeutic gene to specific cells or tissues. This precise control minimizes off-target effects and ensures therapeutic efficacy. Furthermore, researchers often incorporate safety features into the therapeutic gene, such as suicide genes or regulatory elements that allow for the controlled termination of gene expression. This level of precise genetic manipulation allows the creation of highly targeted and controllable therapies. Moreover, continuous research seeks to enhance the longevity and stability of gene expression, aiming for long-lasting therapeutic benefit and potentially eliminating the need for repeated treatments. The development of advanced gene editing tools, such as CRISPR-Cas systems, is further revolutionizing the process, facilitating more precise modifications of the therapeutic gene and further reducing off-target effects. The successful clinical translation of gene therapy requires meticulous planning and execution. The design of clinical trials must carefully consider patient selection criteria to ensure that the therapy is applied to appropriate candidates and to monitor potential adverse events effectively. Rigorous safety monitoring protocols are essential to detect and manage any complications promptly. These protocols typically include regular blood tests, imaging scans, and assessments of clinical symptoms. Data analysis must be carefully conducted to assess the efficacy and safety of the therapy, including evaluating the duration of therapeutic effect, the presence of adverse reactions, and the long-term impact on patients' overall health. Regulatory agencies, like the FDA in the United States and the EMA in Europe, play a crucial role in overseeing the entire process, ensuring the safety and efficacy of gene therapies before they are widely available. The regulatory pathways are stringent, involving preclinical studies, extensive clinical trials, and post-market surveillance, designed to protect patient safety while fostering innovation. Collaboration between scientists, clinicians, regulatory agencies, and ethical review boards is essential for responsible development and application of these transformative therapies.

3.1 Viral Vector Delivery

Viral vectors are essential tools in gene therapy, acting as delivery vehicles for therapeutic genetic material. Their ability to infect specific cell types, coupled with their inherent mechanisms for DNA or RNA delivery, makes them invaluable. However, choosing the right vector is crucial, as each type presents unique advantages and disadvantages. Careful consideration of target cells, the size of the therapeutic gene, and the desired expression duration all inform this critical decision.

Adeno-associated viruses (AAVs) are widely used due to their low immunogenicity and broad tropism, meaning they can infect a wide range of cell types. Their relatively small packaging capacity, however, limits the size of the therapeutic gene that can be delivered. This limitation necessitates careful gene design, often involving the use of smaller, optimized versions of therapeutic genes. For instance, researchers might employ codon optimization to reduce the gene's size without sacrificing protein expression. Strategies like this have improved efficacy and broadened AAV's applicability, even as challenges concerning packaging capacity persist.

Lentiviruses, a class of retroviruses, possess a significant advantage: their ability to integrate their genetic payload into the host cell's genome. This leads to stable, long-term gene expression, a highly sought-after characteristic in gene therapy. However, the risk of insertional mutagenesis, the disruption of a critical gene through random integration, is a significant concern. Rigorous safety testing and the development of improved targeting strategies are therefore paramount. For example, scientists are actively researching ways to direct lentiviral integration to specific, safe genomic locations.

Adenoviruses, known for their high infection efficiency, are another option. They are attractive for their large packaging capacity allowing the delivery of larger genes or multiple genes simultaneously. Unfortunately, their strong immunogenicity – the tendency to trigger a robust immune response – poses a significant challenge. This immune response can lead to inflammation, limiting the duration of therapeutic effect and potentially causing adverse reactions in patients. The transient nature of adenoviral gene expression, stemming from this immune response, often requires multiple administrations to maintain efficacy.

Retroviruses, similar to lentiviruses, offer the capacity for stable gene integration. While they are effective, their tropism is more restricted than AAVs, and safety concerns surrounding insertional mutagenesis remain relevant. Despite these limitations, their strengths in delivering substantial genetic cargo to target cells make them still valuable in specific therapeutic contexts. Continuous refinement and targeted engineering of retroviral vectors are essential for maximizing efficacy while mitigating potential risks.

The selection of a viral vector is a complex process, necessitating an in-depth understanding of the target disease, the desired therapeutic outcome, and the potential risks associated with each vector type. Careful consideration must be given to the vector's packaging capacity, tropism, immunogenicity, and the potential for insertional mutagenesis. Future advancements in vector engineering, including the development of safer and more efficient vectors, will further enhance the power and safety of gene therapy. This is a rapidly evolving field, and staying abreast of the latest research is vital for anyone involved in gene therapy development or clinical application. Continuous innovation in vector design, coupled with advances in gene editing techniques, holds the key to unlock the full therapeutic potential of gene therapy.

Choosing the optimal viral vector requires a thorough understanding of the specific needs of the gene therapy application. Factors such as the target cell type, the size of the therapeutic gene, the desired duration of expression, and the patient's immune status must all be considered. In some cases, a combination of vectors or a combination of viral and non-viral methods might prove optimal, especially in cases of complex genetic diseases or large therapeutic genes. The field is constantly advancing, with new vector types and modifications being developed regularly. Therefore, continuous learning and adaptation to new findings are critical for staying at the forefront of this transformative field. This multifaceted approach, combining deep knowledge of viral vectors with advancements in gene editing techniques, will pave the way for truly impactful personalized medicine and therapeutic treatments. Thorough pre-clinical and clinical testing protocols are crucial. Rigorous testing is essential to ensure safety and effectiveness, balancing the potential benefits against the risks.

3.2 Non-Viral Delivery Methods

Several non-viral methods offer alternative pathways for delivering therapeutic genes, each with its own set of advantages and disadvantages. These methods circumvent some of the limitations associated with viral vectors, such as immunogenicity and insertional mutagenesis, making them attractive alternatives, particularly for certain applications.

Lipid-based nanoparticles, for example, are extensively researched. They encapsulate genetic material, protecting it from degradation and facilitating cellular uptake. The composition of these nanoparticles, including the type of lipid and the presence of targeting ligands, can be meticulously tailored to enhance their delivery efficiency to specific cell types or tissues. This precision targeting minimizes off-target effects, a significant advantage over less specific delivery systems. However, optimizing the formulation for different genes and target tissues remains a challenge, demanding careful consideration of factors such as particle size, surface charge, and stability in physiological environments. Further research is needed to improve their long-term stability and efficacy in vivo.

Another promising approach utilizes physical methods, specifically electroporation. This technique uses brief electrical pulses to create transient pores in cell membranes, allowing the entry of therapeutic DNA or RNA. Electroporation's simplicity and versatility are attractive features; it can be applied in vivo or ex vivo, making it adaptable to a wide range of therapeutic applications. Clinical trials using this method are ongoing, showcasing its potential for gene therapy. However, its efficacy can vary depending on factors such as pulse parameters, cell type, and the physical characteristics of the delivered genetic material. Furthermore, the potential for cell damage and tissue trauma needs careful consideration, requiring careful optimization of electroporation parameters to minimize adverse effects.

Polymer-based delivery systems offer yet another avenue for non-viral gene transfer. Synthetic polymers, specifically designed to encapsulate and protect the therapeutic genetic material, can be engineered to enhance cellular uptake and intracellular trafficking. The biodegradability and biocompatibility of these polymers are crucial for their safety profile. However, ensuring efficient release of the therapeutic gene within the target cell while maintaining the integrity of the polymer remains an ongoing area of active research. Controlling the release kinetics is critical to achieving sustained therapeutic effects without causing toxicity. The development of novel biodegradable polymers with enhanced delivery capabilities is crucial for expanding the therapeutic potential of this approach.

Lastly, the use of hydrodynamic injection offers a unique method for delivering large quantities of genetic material into the liver. This technique involves rapidly injecting a high volume of DNA solution into the circulatory system, forcing the DNA into hepatocytes. While efficient in delivering DNA to the liver, its invasive nature limits its applicability to other tissues and organs. Furthermore, the transient expression of the therapeutic gene may necessitate repeated injections, limiting its long-term effectiveness. Nonetheless, hydrodynamic injection remains a valuable tool, particularly for preclinical studies exploring the therapeutic potential of new genes.

In conclusion, while viral vectors have been the mainstay of gene therapy, non-viral methods provide valuable alternatives with distinct advantages. Further research and development are essential to optimize these techniques and to broaden their clinical applications. Ongoing efforts focus on enhancing their efficiency, specificity, and safety profiles, paving the way for more effective and broadly applicable gene therapies. The choice of delivery method will ultimately depend on the specific therapeutic goal, the target tissue, and the characteristics of the therapeutic gene. A comprehensive understanding of the strengths and limitations of each method is crucial for translating gene therapy advancements into effective clinical treatments. The field is dynamic, and continued innovation will undoubtedly yield even more refined and effective non-viral gene delivery strategies in the future.

4 Addressing Genetic Diseases

Inherited metabolic disorders, a significant class of genetic diseases, present a compelling target for gene editing. These conditions, stemming from defects in enzymes crucial for metabolism, often lead to a buildup of toxic substances or deficiencies in essential compounds. Gene editing offers the potential to correct the underlying genetic defect, restoring normal enzyme function and alleviating the disease's devastating effects. For instance, phenylketonuria (PKU), caused by a deficiency in phenylalanine hydroxylase, is a prime candidate for gene therapy, with ongoing clinical trials exploring the efficacy of various gene editing approaches, targeting the delivery of functional copies of the gene to affected cells. The precise and targeted nature of tools like CRISPR-Cas9 allows for the correction of the faulty gene, avoiding the broader, less precise effects of previous gene therapy methods. Success in these trials could dramatically improve the lives of individuals affected by this debilitating condition.

Monogenic diseases, those caused by a single gene mutation, represent another significant area where gene editing technologies show promise. Cystic fibrosis, a debilitating disease affecting the lungs and other organs, exemplifies this category. The CFTR gene mutation underlies this disease; gene editing offers the potential to correct this mutation directly within affected cells, thereby restoring normal CFTR protein function. While challenges remain, including efficient gene delivery to the relevant lung cells, and potential off-target effects, the potential benefits are immense. Early clinical trials using CRISPR-Cas9 technology demonstrate encouraging signs, showing improvements in lung function and reduced disease severity in some patients, demonstrating the considerable advancements in the field of targeted genome modification.

Hematological disorders, affecting blood cells, offer particularly accessible targets for gene editing due to the ability to isolate and manipulate blood cells ex vivo. Sickle cell disease, a devastating condition characterized by abnormally shaped red blood cells, is a leading example. Gene editing techniques, including CRISPR-Cas9, have shown remarkable success in correcting the underlying genetic defect in blood stem cells. These edited cells can then be transplanted back into the patient, leading to the production of healthy, normally functioning red blood cells. While challenges such as the potential for immune rejection and the need for efficient gene editing remain, the field continues to see significant progress; more clinical trials are expanding access to this life-altering therapy.

Neurological diseases, often characterized by complex genetic underpinnings and challenging accessibility of affected tissues, present a greater hurdle. However, ongoing research is exploring novel gene editing approaches for neurological conditions like Huntington's disease. Though correcting the mutation in the brain remains incredibly complex due to the blood-brain barrier's protection and the sheer number of neurons involved, research focused on gene editing strategies may offer treatments for milder forms or perhaps even preventative measures in at-risk individuals. The development of advanced delivery systems that can effectively target neurons is a significant area of focus, potentially revolutionizing the treatment landscape for these complex conditions.

Cardiovascular diseases, encompassing a wide spectrum of conditions, are also being explored through the lens of gene editing. While the vast majority of cardiovascular diseases are polygenic, with contributions from multiple genes and environmental factors, there are some monogenic forms that are ideal candidates. Research is focused on the development of gene-editing therapies capable of modifying genes associated with familial hypercholesterolemia, a severe form of high cholesterol with life-threatening consequences. By correcting the underlying genetic defect, these therapies aim to reduce cholesterol levels and prevent the development of cardiovascular complications. Early-stage research shows exciting progress but highlights the need for careful long-term safety monitoring.

The application of gene editing to address these diverse categories of genetic diseases showcases its incredible potential to transform medicine. However, it is crucial to acknowledge the challenges that remain, which include off-target effects, immune responses, and the complexities of delivering gene editing tools to specific cell types. Ongoing research continues to address these challenges, refining existing techniques, and developing novel approaches. The careful consideration of ethical implications and the establishment of robust regulatory frameworks are also essential to ensuring that the immense potential of gene editing is harnessed responsibly and equitably.

4.1 Inherited Metabolic Disorders

Inherited metabolic disorders represent a significant challenge in the field of medicine. These conditions, stemming from defects in genes encoding enzymes or transporters crucial for metabolism, lead to the accumulation of harmful substances or deficiencies in essential metabolites. The consequences can range from mild developmental delays to severe, life-threatening complications. Early diagnosis is paramount, allowing for timely intervention and improving quality of life. However, current treatments are often limited, highlighting the urgent need for innovative therapeutic approaches.

Gene editing technologies offer a promising avenue for treating these disorders. Imagine a future where the faulty gene causing a metabolic disorder could be precisely corrected, restoring normal metabolic function and preventing disease progression. This is the potential that gene editing holds. Techniques like CRISPR-Cas9, with its remarkable precision and efficiency, allow researchers to target specific genes, making corrections at the DNA level with increased accuracy. The ability to directly modify the genetic code responsible for metabolic dysregulation holds the key to transformative therapeutic strategies.

A key challenge in treating inherited metabolic disorders is the delivery of the gene-editing machinery to the relevant cells. Viral vectors, particularly adeno-associated viruses (AAVs), have shown promise in delivering gene-editing components to target tissues. Their ability to efficiently transduce cells makes them attractive tools for therapeutic gene editing. However, limitations remain, such as immune responses to viral vectors and the potential for insertional mutagenesis. Continued research aims to overcome these hurdles and develop safer and more effective delivery systems, including exploring the potential of non-viral methods such as lipid nanoparticles and electroporation. These approaches may offer a reduction in immune-related side effects. The optimization of delivery strategies is critical for the successful translation of gene-editing therapies from the laboratory to the clinic.

The complexity of many metabolic pathways poses another significant hurdle. Metabolic disorders often involve multiple genes and pathways, creating a challenging landscape for gene editing. A single gene defect can trigger a cascade of downstream consequences, making it crucial to understand the intricate interactions within the metabolic network. Moreover, the timing of gene editing interventions is critical. Early intervention may be more effective in preventing irreversible damage, but the optimal window of opportunity remains an area of active investigation for each specific disorder. This complex interplay of genes and pathways highlights the need for sophisticated modeling and in-depth understanding of the disease mechanisms.

Developing effective gene editing strategies necessitates careful consideration of off-target effects – unintended modifications to the genome. These off-target effects could lead to unforeseen consequences, potentially exacerbating the condition or even inducing new ones. Rigorous testing and development of refined gene editing tools are necessary to minimize these risks. Furthermore, long-term follow-up studies are essential to monitor the safety and efficacy of gene editing therapies. Understanding potential long-term effects is crucial for responsible and effective clinical application.

Beyond the technical challenges, ethical considerations are paramount. Ensuring equitable access to these potentially life-changing therapies is a critical societal responsibility. The cost of gene editing therapies, coupled with potential challenges in manufacturing and distribution, necessitates careful planning and collaboration to ensure that the benefits reach all populations in need. Furthermore, addressing ethical dilemmas surrounding germline editing, which would alter the genetic makeup of future generations, warrants thoughtful discussion and transparent decision-making processes involving diverse stakeholders. These ethical considerations need careful thought and debate.

Despite these challenges, the potential of gene editing to revolutionize the treatment of inherited metabolic disorders is immense. The ability to directly correct the genetic defects underlying these diseases offers a paradigm shift in therapeutic strategies. Researchers are making significant progress in refining gene editing technologies and developing more effective delivery systems. Addressing the challenges related to off-target effects, long-term safety, and equitable access will be crucial to translating the promise of gene editing into tangible benefits for patients with inherited metabolic disorders. The future holds enormous potential for transforming the lives of countless individuals.

4.2 Monogenic Diseases

Monogenic diseases, caused by a single gene defect, represent a significant target for gene editing therapies. Understanding their underlying mechanisms is crucial for developing effective treatments. These diseases, encompassing a wide range of conditions affecting various organ systems, often manifest with severe and debilitating symptoms, highlighting the urgent need for innovative therapeutic approaches. Many monogenic diseases have a predictable inheritance pattern, making genetic counseling and early diagnosis important for family planning and disease management.

The complexity of monogenic diseases varies significantly, depending on the specific gene affected and the nature of the mutation. Some monogenic disorders are caused by loss-of-function mutations, where the gene fails to produce a functional protein. Other mutations might result in a gain of toxic function, where the altered protein disrupts cellular processes. Still others lead to a change in protein regulation, impacting the timing and level of protein expression.

For example, cystic fibrosis, a classic monogenic disorder, arises from mutations in the CFTR gene, resulting in faulty chloride ion transport across cell membranes. This dysfunction leads to the characteristic mucus buildup in the lungs and other organs. Gene editing strategies for cystic fibrosis aim to correct the underlying genetic defect, restoring CFTR function and alleviating the disease symptoms. The development of specific gene editing tools and delivery systems is critical to successfully targeting the lung cells which are crucial to restoring function and improving patients' quality of life.

Huntington's disease, another example, is a devastating neurodegenerative disorder caused by a trinucleotide repeat expansion in the HTT gene. This expansion leads to the production of a mutant huntingtin protein, which accumulates in brain cells and causes neuronal dysfunction and cell death. Gene editing approaches for Huntington's disease might focus on reducing the expression of the mutant huntingtin protein or correcting the underlying genetic defect itself. While challenges remain, preclinical studies show promising approaches, suggesting the potential of gene editing to provide some relief or even prevent disease progression.

However, the application of gene editing to monogenic diseases is not without its obstacles. One major challenge is the delivery of gene editing tools to the target cells and tissues. Many diseases affect specific cell types within organs or tissues, presenting a significant hurdle for effective delivery. Furthermore, the efficiency of gene editing can vary depending on the target gene, the type of mutation, and the gene editing technology used. Off-target effects, unintended edits to the genome, pose another critical concern, and careful optimization and quality control are necessary to ensure safety and therapeutic efficacy. Moreover, the long-term effects of gene editing therapies remain largely unknown, requiring rigorous long-term follow-up studies to monitor potential adverse events. The ethical considerations surrounding gene editing, particularly in germline cells, necessitate careful consideration of the societal impact of these technologies. Access and equity issues surrounding advanced gene therapies present additional challenges; these highly specialized treatments often come with significant costs. Addressing these obstacles through further research and careful planning is crucial for realizing the full therapeutic potential of gene editing in monogenic diseases.

Despite these challenges, the field of gene editing offers significant promise for treating monogenic diseases. The ability to precisely correct or modify the underlying genetic defect represents a paradigm shift in therapeutic strategies, potentially offering lasting cures rather than only managing symptoms. Ongoing research continues to refine gene editing technologies and delivery methods, paving the way for safer and more effective treatments. Improvements in CRISPR-Cas systems and advancements in delivery methods, such as viral and non-viral vectors, are continually improving the possibilities for treating a greater range of these diseases.

The future of monogenic disease treatment may involve individualized approaches, tailoring gene editing strategies to specific mutations and patient characteristics. Advances in our understanding of disease pathogenesis and genetic modifiers could also enhance the precision and effectiveness of gene editing therapies. A multifaceted approach, combining gene editing with other therapeutic strategies, holds the potential to provide comprehensive disease management and enhance patient outcomes, moving beyond symptomatic relief to effective, potentially curative treatments for monogenic diseases. As research continues, a brighter future emerges for those affected by these debilitating conditions.

4.3 Hematological Disorders

Hematological disorders, encompassing a wide spectrum of blood-related diseases, represent a significant area where gene editing technologies hold immense promise. Conditions like sickle cell anemia, -thalassemia, and various leukemias stem from genetic defects affecting blood cell production, function, or both. These diseases often lead to chronic pain, organ damage, and significantly reduced life expectancy. Gene editing offers a potential pathway towards curative therapies, targeting the underlying genetic mutations to restore normal blood cell function. The application of CRISPR-Cas systems, for example, has shown remarkable success in preclinical models of sickle cell disease. Scientists have successfully corrected the faulty -globin gene in hematopoietic stem cells (HSCs), the precursors of all blood cells. After gene correction and transplantation of these modified HSCs, animal models exhibited a substantial reduction in sickle cell-related symptoms and an increase in healthy red blood cells. Similar strategies are being explored for -thalassemia, another inherited blood disorder resulting from reduced or absent -globin production. Successful correction of the genetic defect in HSCs could lead to sustained production of functional hemoglobin, alleviating the need for lifelong blood transfusions and reducing the risk of complications.

However, the clinical translation of gene editing for hematological disorders faces substantial challenges. One key obstacle is the efficient delivery of the gene editing machinery to the target cells. While viral vectors, such as lentiviruses and adeno-associated viruses (AAVs), are commonly used, their limitations include insertional mutagenesis and potential immunogenicity. Non-viral methods, such as electroporation and lipid nanoparticles, offer alternative approaches but often exhibit lower efficiency. Furthermore, ensuring precise targeting of the gene editing machinery is crucial to avoid off-target effects, which could have detrimental consequences. Rigorous quality control and careful monitoring are essential to minimize unintended edits to the genome and ensure the safety of gene-edited cells.

Another hurdle lies in the efficient expansion and engraftment of gene-edited HSCs. Successful transplantation requires a sufficient number of modified HSCs to engraft in the bone marrow and generate a therapeutic level of corrected blood cells. Optimization of culture conditions and the development of novel selection strategies to enrich for gene-edited cells are crucial steps toward achieving efficient engraftment. The long-term persistence and stability of gene correction are also critical considerations. While early clinical trials have shown promising results, long-term follow-up studies are necessary to assess the durability of the therapeutic effect and to monitor for potential late-onset complications.

Beyond single-gene disorders, gene editing technologies are also being investigated for the treatment of hematological malignancies, such as acute lymphoblastic leukemia (ALL) and multiple myeloma. These cancers are characterized by uncontrolled proliferation of abnormal blood cells. Gene editing approaches aim to either eliminate cancerous cells or to modify them to render them susceptible to targeted therapies. For instance, researchers are exploring the use of CRISPR-Cas systems to disrupt genes critical for cancer cell survival or to enhance the efficacy of immunotherapies by engineering T cells to specifically target cancer cells. These strategies are still in early stages of development, but they hold tremendous potential for improving the treatment outcomes of these life-threatening diseases. Careful planning, including stringent safety protocols, robust quality control, and long-term monitoring, will be crucial for successful clinical translation. Furthermore, a thorough understanding of the underlying mechanisms involved in the pathogenesis of hematological malignancies will enhance the design and effectiveness of gene-editing strategies.

The ethical considerations surrounding the use of gene editing in hematological disorders require careful deliberation. While gene editing offers the potential for curative therapies, it also raises concerns about the long-term consequences of genetic modifications and the potential for unintended off-target effects. Rigorous preclinical studies and carefully designed clinical trials are essential to ensure the safety and efficacy of these treatments. Equitable access to gene editing therapies is also a critical consideration, ensuring that these advanced treatments are available to all patients in need, regardless of socioeconomic background or geographical location. Transparency and public engagement are key in navigating this complex and rapidly evolving field, fostering responsible innovation while safeguarding patient welfare and societal well-being. The ongoing advancements in gene editing technologies, coupled with a focus on addressing the existing challenges, promise a future where many life-threatening hematological disorders can be effectively treated or even cured.

4.4 Neurological Diseases

Neurological diseases represent a significant challenge in the field of gene therapy, encompassing a vast spectrum of disorders affecting the brain, spinal cord, and peripheral nerves. Conditions like Huntington's disease, Parkinson's disease, Alzheimer's disease, and amyotrophic lateral sclerosis (ALS) stem from complex genetic underpinnings, posing unique hurdles for gene-editing interventions. The intricate structure of the nervous system, the presence of the blood-brain barrier, and the long lifespan of neurons all contribute to the difficulties encountered in achieving effective gene delivery and therapeutic outcomes.
Targeting specific genes implicated in neurological disorders is a complex endeavor. Many diseases result from a multitude of genetic variations, not just single gene mutations. Even in monogenic diseases like Huntington's disease, where a single

gene's mutation is the primary cause, delivering a therapeutic gene to a sufficient number of affected neurons to halt disease progression presents a considerable obstacle. Precise targeting and efficient delivery mechanisms are paramount, requiring a delicate balance between efficacy and safety.

The blood-brain barrier acts as a protective shield, preventing many substances from entering the brain. This barrier significantly limits the effectiveness of gene therapy approaches that rely on systemic delivery. Scientists are actively exploring various methods to circumvent this limitation, including the use of targeted viral vectors specifically engineered to penetrate the blood-brain barrier or the development of non-viral delivery systems with enhanced brain-targeting capabilities. Nanotechnology-based approaches, such as liposomes and exosomes, are gaining attention for their potential to deliver therapeutic genes across the blood-brain barrier. Careful consideration of vector choice, dose, and route of administration is crucial in optimizing delivery strategies.

Beyond delivery challenges, the long lifespan of neurons presents another major obstacle. Therapeutic gene correction might need to be sustained for many years, if not a lifetime, to provide lasting clinical benefit. Integrating the therapeutic gene into the neuronal genome is a potential solution to ensure long-term expression. However, random integration could carry risks of insertional mutagenesis, potentially causing unintended side effects. Scientists are actively researching strategies to precisely target the therapeutic gene integration into specific safe sites within the genome to mitigate these risks.

Further complicating the treatment of neurological diseases, the high degree of genetic and phenotypic heterogeneity adds to the complexity of developing effective gene therapies. The same disease can manifest differently in individuals due to genetic background, environmental factors, and epigenetic modifications. This requires a more personalized approach, focusing on tailoring treatments to each patient's unique genetic profile and disease progression. Precision medicine and strategies that account for genetic variation are critical to improve the chances of successful treatment.

Moreover, ethical considerations surrounding neurological disease gene therapy warrant careful consideration. The potential for off-target effects, the long-term consequences of gene editing, and the potential for misuse of these technologies require robust ethical frameworks and regulatory guidelines. Extensive preclinical research and meticulously designed clinical trials are essential to ensure patient safety and to gather the necessary data to fully understand the long-term risks and benefits. Open communication with patients, and ongoing monitoring of outcomes, are crucial in establishing public trust and building confidence in this rapidly advancing field. The development of improved diagnostic tools and biomarkers are paramount to track disease progression and ensure a more precise assessment of treatment efficacy.

Despite these challenges, significant advancements are being made in gene editing technologies for neurological diseases. CRISPR-Cas systems, particularly, have shown promise for correcting gene mutations involved in several neurological disorders. Ongoing research focuses on optimizing the precision and efficiency of these systems while mitigating potential off-target effects. Developing improved delivery methods, designing safer vectors, and performing extensive preclinical research and clinical trials will be critical in advancing the field and translating these promising technologies into effective therapies. The potential to alleviate the suffering associated with these devastating diseases warrants a concerted effort from researchers, clinicians, and regulatory agencies to overcome the significant hurdles involved.

The future of gene editing for neurological diseases lies in the development of novel, more effective strategies for precise gene targeting, efficient delivery across the blood-brain barrier, and sustained therapeutic gene expression. Close collaboration between geneticists, neuroscientists, clinicians, and bioengineers will accelerate the development of new therapies, opening avenues for improved diagnosis, effective treatment options, and hopefully cures for some of the most challenging neurological disorders. The potential benefits are vast, but navigating the complex ethical and technological challenges involved remains crucial for responsible and effective advancement in this field. A multi-pronged approach that addresses delivery, safety, efficacy, and the ethical considerations will be essential to realizing the full potential of gene editing in addressing neurological diseases and improving the quality of life for affected individuals.

4.5 Cardiovascular Diseases

Cardiovascular diseases represent a significant global health burden, claiming millions of lives annually. The complexity of these diseases, often involving multiple genes and environmental factors, presents a considerable challenge for traditional therapeutic approaches. However, gene editing technologies offer a potential paradigm shift, providing unprecedented opportunities for both prevention and treatment.

One promising avenue lies in targeting genes associated with familial hypercholesterolemia (FH), a heritable disorder leading to high LDL cholesterol levels and increased risk of heart attacks and strokes. Gene editing could potentially correct the genetic defect responsible for FH, thus lowering cholesterol levels and mitigating the associated risks. Studies utilizing CRISPR-Cas9 have shown encouraging results in preclinical models, with successful modification of the PCSK9 gene, a key regulator of LDL cholesterol metabolism. While still in early stages, these advancements suggest the potential for a curative approach to FH.

Beyond FH, gene editing holds potential for treating other cardiovascular disorders. For example, inherited cardiomyopathies, characterized by weakened or thickened heart muscle, often result from mutations in genes encoding cardiac structural proteins. Correcting these mutations via gene editing could potentially restore normal heart function and improve patient outcomes. However, the challenges in efficiently delivering the gene-editing machinery to the heart muscle, along with the potential for off-target effects, necessitate careful consideration and further research.

Atherosclerosis, the underlying cause of most cardiovascular diseases, is a complex process involving inflammation, cholesterol deposition, and plaque formation within blood vessels. Gene editing strategies could be employed to modulate the expression of genes involved in these processes. For instance, targeting genes that regulate inflammation could potentially reduce plaque formation and stabilize existing plaques, thus reducing the risk of heart attacks and strokes. Research into this area is still in its infancy, but the potential to alter the disease trajectory is substantial.

Furthermore, gene editing's impact extends beyond the treatment of individual diseases. It could also play a pivotal role in developing novel diagnostic tools. The ability to precisely edit specific genomic sequences can be harnessed to create highly sensitive and specific genetic markers for cardiovascular risk assessment. Such markers could allow for early detection and personalized preventative strategies, significantly improving patient prognosis. This preventative application is crucial, as early intervention can significantly impact disease progression and long-term health.

The field, however, is not without its challenges. Delivering the gene editing machinery to the relevant cells in the cardiovascular system efficiently and safely presents a major hurdle. Furthermore, the potential for off-target effects – unintended edits to the genome – remains a significant concern. Thorough preclinical studies and robust safety protocols are essential to mitigate these risks. Moreover, ethical considerations surrounding the use of gene editing technologies in cardiovascular disease require careful deliberation and societal consensus. Transparency in research and open dialogue with stakeholders are paramount to ensure responsible implementation.

The translation of gene editing technologies into effective cardiovascular therapies requires a multidisciplinary approach. Collaboration between geneticists, cardiologists, bioengineers, and clinicians is crucial to overcome the technical and ethical challenges involved. Rigorous clinical trials are needed to evaluate the safety and efficacy of these novel therapies, ensuring that they are both effective and accessible to patients who stand to benefit. The development of standardized protocols for gene editing procedures is also vital for widespread adoption and consistent outcomes. The potential benefits are profound, but only with careful and responsible implementation can we harness the transformative power of gene editing for cardiovascular health.

5 Ethical and Societal Implications

Germline editing, the modification of genes in reproductive cells, presents profound ethical challenges. Altering the human germline has the potential to introduce changes that are heritable, affecting not only the individual treated but also all their future descendants. This raises concerns about unforeseen consequences and the potential for unintended harm across generations. The long-term effects of such modifications are largely unknown, introducing significant uncertainty into the equation. Ethical frameworks must grapple with the responsibility we bear towards future generations and the potential for irreversible alterations to the human gene pool. The principle of non-maleficence, the obligation to do no harm, is especially crucial here, demanding careful consideration and stringent safety protocols. The potential for misuse, such as creating 'designer babies' with enhanced traits, further complicates the matter, demanding robust regulatory oversight and societal consensus.

Questions of equitable access to gene editing technologies also demand urgent attention. The high cost of gene editing therapies could exacerbate existing health disparities, leaving vulnerable populations without access to potentially life-saving treatments. This raises crucial questions about justice and fairness in healthcare. A global commitment to equitable distribution of benefits, perhaps involving international collaborations and philanthropic initiatives, is essential to ensure that these powerful technologies don't widen the gap between the haves and the have-nots. Failure to address this inequity would risk creating a two-tiered system of healthcare, further marginalizing disadvantaged communities. Developing sustainable models for equitable access requires careful planning, resource allocation, and ongoing dialogue with affected populations.

The potential societal impact of gene editing extends beyond individual health. Broader societal implications need careful consideration. Changes to the human gene pool could have unforeseen consequences for human evolution and biodiversity. The potential for unintended ecological effects, resulting from the introduction of novel genetic traits into populations, must be examined. Moreover, societal anxieties surrounding genetic enhancement could lead to widespread social discrimination or stigmatization of individuals with particular genetic profiles. These far-reaching implications necessitate open and inclusive public dialogue to establish shared values and guidelines governing the responsible development and application of this technology. These discussions must involve experts from diverse fields, including ethicists, social scientists, policymakers, and the general public, ensuring a multifaceted approach to navigating these complex issues.

Responsible innovation requires a multi-pronged approach. It necessitates the development of rigorous safety standards and regulatory frameworks, informed by ethical principles and ongoing scientific research. Transparency in research, open communication with the public, and proactive engagement with ethical concerns are vital. International collaboration is essential to establish globally harmonized regulations and guidelines, preventing a fragmented approach that could allow for the exploitation of regulatory loopholes. Strengthening ethical review boards and promoting robust public education are key to ensuring responsible development and use of this powerful technology. Only through this comprehensive approach can we hope to harness the therapeutic potential of gene editing while mitigating its associated risks and ethical dilemmas. The future application of gene editing hinges on a proactive, ethical, and equitable approach.

Addressing the ethical and societal implications of gene editing is not a task for scientists alone; it necessitates a broad, collaborative effort. Policymakers must create robust regulatory frameworks that balance innovation with ethical considerations and societal values. Educators have a crucial role in shaping public understanding of gene editing and its potential impact. Open and honest public discourse is vital to building a shared understanding and forming a societal consensus on the appropriate use of these powerful technologies. Engaging religious, philosophical, and cultural perspectives will enrich the dialogue and ensure a diverse range of viewpoints are considered. Ultimately, the future of gene editing relies on a collective commitment to responsible innovation, equity, and ethical leadership. This responsibility rests upon the shoulders of scientists, policymakers, and individuals alike, requiring collaborative effort and informed decisions to shape a future where gene editing benefits humanity as a whole.

5.1 Germline Editing Concerns

Germline editing, altering the genes passed from parents to offspring, presents unique ethical and societal challenges. Unlike somatic cell editing, which affects only the individual, germline modifications are heritable, impacting future generations. This raises concerns about unintended consequences that could ripple through populations, affecting individuals who never consented to such genetic alterations. The potential for unforeseen health problems, both immediate and long-term, across multiple generations, remains a significant unknown. Scientists must fully grasp the ramifications of such powerful tools before widespread application can be considered. Careful, comprehensive research is crucial to fully understand the potential risks and to develop robust safety protocols.

The potential for unintended consequences extends beyond individual health. Germline editing could inadvertently alter human evolution in unpredictable ways. We lack a complete understanding of gene interactions and the complex interplay of genes and environment. Altering even a single gene could have cascading effects on other genes and traits, leading to unforeseen and potentially detrimental evolutionary outcomes. The complexity of the human genome and the limitations of our current knowledge necessitates extreme caution when considering changes that affect the entirety of a human's genetic makeup. Long-term studies spanning generations will be crucial to assess these risks adequately.

Another significant concern revolves around the equitable access to germline editing technologies. If these technologies become a reality, ensuring equitable distribution will be paramount. Without careful consideration, the ability to enhance human traits through germline editing may exacerbate existing social inequalities. Wealthy individuals and nations might have preferential access to these technologies, leading to a widening gap between the "genetically enhanced" and the rest of the population. A fair and just system for allocating access to this technology, if it is deemed safe and appropriate, is absolutely critical. We must avoid the creation of a genetic divide that amplifies societal disparities, even if the initial intention behind these therapies is to reduce them.

The ethical implications extend beyond potential health risks and access issues. The prospect of "designer babies" raises profound philosophical and moral questions. The idea of choosing specific traits for our children—such as intelligence, physical appearance, or disease resistance—raises complex questions about parental autonomy and the value of human diversity. Society needs a broad and inclusive discussion to define the acceptable boundaries of genetic modification. What constitutes a permissible modification versus a harmful or unethical one? These discussions are necessary to guide policy and regulation surrounding the use of this powerful technology, to ensure it is used responsibly and ethically. It is imperative to weigh potential benefits carefully against the profound and potentially irreversible consequences.

Furthermore, the potential for misuse of germline editing technologies is another significant area of concern. These technologies could be used not only for therapeutic purposes but also for non-therapeutic enhancement, potentially leading to an arms race in genetic modification. This could create a situation where the competitive pressure to enhance human traits is overwhelming, leading to a potentially unethical and harmful arms race, much like that associated with nuclear weapons. This arms race will have to be mitigated, and international regulation and strict ethical frameworks are crucial to prevent the misuse of such powerful technology and safeguard future generations. It's critical to maintain focus on human well-being and ethical considerations, while avoiding a purely competitive enhancement-focused agenda.

In conclusion, the potential benefits of germline editing are undoubtedly substantial, especially concerning the eradication of inheritable diseases. However, the ethical and societal implications are too profound to ignore. Thorough and transparent discussions involving scientists, ethicists, policymakers, and the public are vital before such technologies are used clinically. A cautious and incremental approach, coupled with a robust ethical framework, is essential to harness the power of germline editing responsibly, ensuring that the benefits reach all populations while mitigating the potential risks for present and future generations. Proactive measures and regulations are vital for preventing the misuse of these technologies and safeguarding ethical principles while promoting human well-being.

5.2 Equity & Access

Ensuring equitable access to gene editing technologies is paramount, a moral imperative demanding immediate attention. The transformative potential of these technologies–to cure diseases, alleviate suffering, and improve lives–must not be confined to the privileged few. We must actively work to dismantle the barriers that prevent widespread access, fostering a future where everyone, regardless of their background or location, can benefit.

This requires a multifaceted approach. Firstly, robust and transparent regulatory frameworks are essential. These frameworks must be designed to balance innovation with safety, ensuring rigorous testing and approval processes without stifling research or hindering access for those who need it most. Overly stringent regulations can inadvertently create monopolies, limiting access rather than expanding it.

Furthermore, substantial investment in research and development is needed, particularly in low\item and middle-income countries (LMICs). This includes funding basic research, training scientists and healthcare professionals, and building the necessary infrastructure. International collaborations are crucial, leveraging the expertise of high-income countries while empowering LMICs to develop their own capacities. The sharing of knowledge, technologies, and resources is not merely an ethical consideration but a strategic necessity.

Beyond funding, educational initiatives play a pivotal role. We need to increase public awareness about gene editing technologies, addressing concerns and misconceptions while highlighting their potential benefits. Effective communication, tailored to diverse audiences, is crucial to build trust and support for responsible innovation. Educational outreach must target both healthcare professionals and the general public, fostering informed decision-making.

Addressing economic disparities is another critical aspect of ensuring equity. The costs associated with gene editing therapies are considerable, potentially creating a significant barrier to access. Innovative financing mechanisms are essential, including the exploration of tiered pricing models, public-private partnerships, and international collaborations to reduce costs and improve affordability. Financial barriers should not determine who benefits from these life-changing technologies.

Geographic disparities also present a major challenge. Access to specialized healthcare facilities and qualified personnel is often limited in many regions of the world. Telemedicine, mobile health technologies, and decentralized healthcare models can help bridge these geographical gaps, bringing advanced therapies to those who currently lack access. Strategic collaborations between healthcare providers and technology companies are necessary for building effective and sustainable solutions.

Finally, ethical considerations must remain central to our efforts. We must prioritize equitable distribution and address potential biases in access. Robust mechanisms for monitoring and evaluating the impact of gene editing technologies on different populations are necessary to identify and rectify any disparities that may arise. This constant vigilance is critical to ensure responsible and equitable deployment of these powerful technologies. The promise of gene editing should benefit humanity as a whole, not just a select few. Active engagement with community leaders, patients, and advocacy groups ensures that decisions reflect the diverse perspectives and needs of all stakeholders. This collaborative approach is vital in ensuring that the benefits of gene editing technologies are accessible to all.

6 Challenges and Future Directions

Off-target effects remain a significant hurdle. While CRISPR-Cas systems offer unprecedented precision, the possibility of unintended edits at other genomic locations persists. These off-target modifications can lead to unforeseen consequences, potentially causing new diseases or exacerbating existing ones. Minimizing these effects requires refining the design of guide RNAs, improving the specificity of Cas enzymes, and developing more sensitive detection methods to identify off-target events. Advanced computational tools and machine learning algorithms are being employed to predict and prevent off-target effects, with the aim of increasing the safety and efficacy of gene editing therapies. Furthermore, novel Cas variants with enhanced specificity are continuously being discovered and engineered, promising a future with significantly reduced off-target activity. This remains a crucial area of active research, demanding constant refinement and innovation.

The body's immune system can mount a significant response against gene editing components. The introduction of foreign genetic material, such as viral vectors or Cas enzymes, can trigger an immune reaction that compromises the effectiveness or safety of the treatment. Immune responses can manifest as inflammation, a reduction in the number of edited cells, or even the development of severe autoimmune disorders. Strategies to mitigate this involve utilizing immunomodulatory agents alongside gene editing therapies to dampen the immune response, employing less immunogenic delivery vehicles, or engineering gene editing components to be less immunogenic themselves. Further research is critical to understanding the mechanisms of these immune responses and to designing effective strategies for their prevention or management. The ultimate goal is to ensure that the body's defense systems don't counteract the intended therapeutic effects.

Long-term consequences of gene editing are largely unknown. While short-term efficacy and safety data are crucial, a comprehensive understanding requires long-term follow-up studies to assess the durability of gene edits and to identify any delayed adverse effects. These studies are inherently challenging, demanding careful patient selection, long-term monitoring, and sophisticated analytical methods. The potential for unforeseen complications, including insertional mutagenesis, epigenetic alterations, or the development of late-onset diseases, necessitates rigorous long-term evaluations before widespread clinical application. Such studies provide invaluable data for improving the long-term safety and efficacy profiles of gene editing interventions, making them safer and more reliable. It requires significant resources and time, but it is absolutely indispensable to ensuring the responsible deployment of this potent technology. Ethical considerations related to informed consent and patient autonomy are paramount, particularly given the potential unknown long-term effects. We need robust frameworks to ensure patient safety and well-being.

Addressing these challenges will require a multidisciplinary approach. Biochemists, geneticists, immunologists, clinicians, and ethicists need to collaborate closely to advance gene editing technologies safely and ethically. Technological improvements, such as enhanced delivery systems, more specific Cas enzymes, and improved screening methods for off-target effects, are crucial. However, these advancements must be coupled with rigorous clinical trials, robust safety monitoring, and a thorough ethical evaluation to ensure that gene editing therapies are implemented responsibly and equitably. Developing regulatory frameworks that balance innovation with patient safety is also essential. International collaboration is needed, to foster innovation, accelerate the development of safer gene therapies, and ensure broad access across the globe. Open data sharing and standardization of protocols will streamline research and ensure consistent quality and safety. The future of gene editing depends on our collective efforts, prioritizing both the power of the technology and the well-being of patients. This collaborative endeavor is crucial for the long-term success and responsible implementation of this ground-breaking field.

6.1 Off-Target Effects

Off-target effects represent a significant hurdle in the widespread clinical application of gene editing technologies. These unintended modifications to the genome can range from subtle alterations in gene expression to large-scale chromosomal rearrangements, potentially leading to unpredictable and harmful consequences for the patient. Minimizing off-target effects is crucial for ensuring the safety and efficacy of gene therapies. Careful experimental design and rigorous quality control are paramount.

Current gene editing tools, while remarkably precise, are not perfect. The inherent limitations of targeting mechanisms, such as CRISPR-Cas systems' occasional binding to unintended DNA sequences, necessitate a multi-pronged approach to mitigation. Researchers are actively exploring strategies to improve target specificity, including the design of improved guide RNAs (gRNAs) with enhanced binding affinity and reduced off-target activity. Computational tools that predict potential off-target sites are also crucial for identifying and avoiding them during experimental design.

Furthermore, advanced bioinformatics techniques play a crucial role in detecting off-target effects. Next-generation sequencing (NGS) technologies allow for comprehensive analysis of the entire genome, identifying any unintended modifications with high sensitivity. The development and implementation of sophisticated algorithms are crucial to accurately and efficiently distinguish off-target events from natural genetic variations. These bioinformatic approaches are vital for the clinical translation of gene editing technologies.

Beyond improved targeting and detection, innovative strategies are being developed to minimize off-target effects directly. One approach involves the development of modified Cas enzymes with enhanced specificity, either through protein engineering or through the use of alternative CRISPR systems with improved fidelity. Another promising strategy involves using multiple gRNAs targeting different regions of the same gene, ensuring that even if an off-target effect occurs at one site, the overall efficiency of the editing process is still high. This redundancy mitigates the risk.

The development of novel delivery systems could also indirectly reduce off-target effects. Precise delivery of editing machinery to target cells would minimize the chance of unintended modifications in other cells or tissues. Improved delivery methods are critical. The reduction of off-target effects depends heavily upon it. By reducing the amount of editing machinery in non-target areas, the number of unintended alterations can be dramatically reduced, thereby improving the overall safety of the therapy.

Evaluating the long-term consequences of off-target effects requires extensive research. Studies in model organisms, as well as carefully designed clinical trials, are essential to assess both short-term and long-term effects of these unintended alterations. This long-term monitoring is crucial for ensuring patient safety and improving our understanding of the overall consequences of gene editing procedures, identifying any late-onset adverse events. Longitudinal studies are integral to safe gene therapy

implementation.
Careful consideration of all potential off-target effects is essential for responsible development and implementation of gene editing therapies. We must balance the potential benefits of these groundbreaking technologies with the risks associated with unintended genomic modifications. This will require collaboration between scientists, clinicians, ethicists, and regulators to establish clear guidelines and safety protocols, carefully weighing risks against potential benefits. Only through such a careful and coordinated effort can we fully realize the potential of gene editing while minimizing the potential harm.
Finally, we must acknowledge that there is no "perfect" solution to completely eliminate off-target effects. Our focus should be on continuously refining our techniques, developing more accurate and efficient methods, and employing rigorous monitoring strategies to detect and mitigate any adverse events. The field of gene editing is constantly evolving, and ongoing research is crucial to address these challenges effectively. Continuous improvement will be critical to reducing the impact of off-target effects and ensuring safer, more effective gene editing therapies.

6.2 Immune Responses

The human immune system, a complex network of cells and proteins, plays a crucial role in recognizing and eliminating foreign substances, including the components used in gene editing therapies. This recognition process can trigger an immune response, potentially hindering the success of the treatment or even causing harmful side effects. Understanding these immune responses is paramount for developing safe and effective gene editing strategies. Different components of the gene editing machinery, such as viral vectors or CRISPR-Cas components themselves, can act as antigens, triggering an immune reaction. Pre-existing immunity to viral vectors, for instance, can limit the effectiveness of gene therapy. This necessitates careful consideration of patient history and the selection of appropriate vectors to minimize this risk. Furthermore, the introduction of foreign genetic material can elicit both innate and adaptive immune responses, and these responses can vary significantly between individuals depending on their genetic background and previous exposure to similar antigens.

Effective gene editing strategies require careful consideration of potential immune responses. Researchers are actively exploring different ways to mitigate these responses, including immunosuppressive drugs or the use of immune-evading vectors. For example, modifications to viral vectors can reduce their immunogenicity, making them less likely to trigger a strong immune reaction. Alternatively, gene editing techniques that utilize non-viral delivery methods, like lipid nanoparticles, might offer advantages in terms of reduced immunogenicity. Ultimately, a deeper understanding of the interactions between gene editing components and the immune system is necessary to refine existing methods and develop novel strategies to circumvent potentially harmful immune responses.

The development of personalized gene editing therapies requires a thorough understanding of individual immune profiles. This includes factors like HLA type, previous infections, and genetic predisposition to autoimmune diseases. Such personalized approaches can significantly improve the safety and efficacy of gene therapies. For example, individuals with pre-existing immunity to a specific viral vector might benefit from a different delivery method or a treatment designed to mitigate the immune reaction. Researchers might develop diagnostic tools to assess individual immune responses and predict the potential for adverse events, allowing for tailored treatment strategies to improve safety and effectiveness. Incorporating this level of precision enhances the likelihood of successful outcomes in patients. Minimizing immune responses is essential for the long-term success of gene editing therapies. Even if an initial treatment is successful, the persistence of edited genetic material could trigger delayed or chronic immune reactions, potentially leading to complications or requiring additional interventions. Chronic inflammation, for example, can contribute to tissue damage and organ dysfunction. Therefore, strategies that limit both the initial and long-term immune responses are crucial for long-term safety and effectiveness of gene therapies. Researchers are actively researching immune-modulating strategies, including the design of immunotolerant gene editing approaches, to promote the long-term integration of edited genetic material without triggering harmful immune reactions.

Beyond viral vectors and CRISPR components, the edited cells themselves can elicit immune responses. The altered expression of proteins or the introduction of novel epitopes can stimulate immune cells, potentially leading to cell destruction or an autoimmune reaction. The careful design of gene editing therapies, coupled with advanced immune monitoring techniques, is essential to detect and manage such responses. Researchers need to understand the specifics of each case, investigating the molecular mechanisms that trigger these immune responses, in order to improve the efficacy and safety of gene therapy protocols and develop better immunomodulatory strategies. Careful monitoring of patients throughout the course of treatment is key for early detection and management of adverse events.

The immune system's complexity presents a significant hurdle for successful gene editing therapies. In addition to adaptive immunity, involving T cells and B cells, the innate immune system, involving macrophages and natural killer cells, can also play a crucial role in recognizing and eliminating gene-edited cells. Understanding both branches of the immune system and their interactions with the gene editing components is vital for developing effective strategies to minimize adverse effects and improve the therapeutic efficacy of gene editing approaches. Advanced approaches that utilize immunomodulatory agents or design genetic edits that reduce immunogenicity are essential in advancing the field of gene editing and bringing this promising technology to the clinic. Moreover, a deeper understanding of this intricate interplay is essential to ensure the safe and effective translation of gene editing technologies into clinical practice, ultimately leading to successful personalized therapies for a wide range of diseases.

The challenge of predicting and managing immune responses remains a major obstacle to the widespread adoption of gene editing therapies. Current research focuses on refining our understanding of the precise mechanisms involved in immune response activation and developing more effective strategies to dampen them. The development of novel methods for delivering genetic material, optimizing the design of gene editing tools, and utilizing immune-modulating agents represents a significant area of ongoing research. These advances are crucial for ensuring the safe and effective translation of gene editing technologies from the laboratory to the clinic. This continuous effort is essential to bring the transformative potential of gene editing to patients while mitigating potential risks.

6.3 Long-Term Effects

The long-term effects of gene editing remain a significant area of investigation, requiring rigorous study and careful monitoring. While the immediate results of gene editing therapies show promise, the potential for unforeseen consequences necessitates extended follow-up in clinical trials and post-market surveillance. This is not simply a matter of observing treatment efficacy; it's about comprehensive assessment encompassing a range of physiological factors, cellular behavior, and potential interactions with the broader biological landscape. We must anticipate and prepare for the possibility of delayed or subtle effects that might not be apparent within the shorter timeframe of typical clinical studies.

Understanding the long-term impact requires a multi-faceted approach. We need to move beyond simply tracking the expression of edited genes and instead focus on how these edits affect overall physiological function over many years. This involves careful examination of potential effects on other genes, on cellular processes, and on the entire organism. It means developing sensitive assays to detect subtle changes, which may only manifest later in life. Such comprehensive longitudinal studies are paramount to assuring the long-term safety and efficacy of these innovative therapies.

For instance, consider the challenges in assessing the long-term effects of gene editing in treating a chronic disease like cystic fibrosis. While immediate improvements in lung function might be observed, the ultimate success of the therapy hinges on whether these improvements are sustained for decades, and if the edited gene remains stable within the patient's genome. The potential for insertional mutagenesis – where the gene editing process inadvertently causes unintended genetic alterations – must also be closely monitored over time. It is crucial to evaluate potential cumulative effects and unforeseen interactions with other genetic and environmental factors.

Moreover, the potential for immune system responses to gene-edited cells is a significant concern that extends beyond the immediate post-treatment period. Long-term monitoring is needed to detect any delayed or chronic inflammatory reactions, which could be triggered by the edited cells, or by the viral vectors used for delivery. This is especially relevant in therapies targeting immune cells, where the treatment itself could modify immune functionality and potentially result in unanticipated effects on immunity to other diseases. Continuous evaluation, incorporating advanced immunological techniques, is essential. Beyond individual patient outcomes, we need to consider the potential impact on subsequent generations, particularly in the context of germline gene editing. While the ethical debates surrounding germline editing are complex and extensive, assessing the long-term ramifications for offspring is paramount. This necessitates rigorous research into multigenerational effects, considering not only the direct impact of the gene edit, but also its potential consequences on gene expression, development, and overall health throughout the lifespan of future generations. Any long-term study plan must carefully incorporate these considerations.

The development of new technologies to assess these long-term impacts is equally crucial. Advances in sequencing technologies allow us to monitor the genome over time with increasing accuracy and efficiency. Sophisticated imaging techniques provide high-resolution views of cellular processes and physiological function. These technological advancements are instrumental to our capacity for effectively tracking and mitigating any long-term effects. Coupled with large-scale clinical trials and comprehensive data collection and analysis, we can build the knowledge base necessary for responsible application of this technology.

Finally, transparency and collaboration are essential. Open data sharing among researchers and regulatory agencies is crucial to accelerating our understanding of long-term effects. International collaborations are necessary to pool resources and share data, thereby expediting the process of evaluating the long-term safety and efficacy of these therapies. Only through this shared commitment to rigorous research and collaboration can we ensure that the promise of gene editing is realized responsibly and safely, for generations to come. This collaborative effort will provide the essential evidence base required to guide responsible regulation and policy.

7 Regulatory Landscape & Safety

Navigating the complex world of gene editing necessitates a thorough understanding of the regulatory landscape and stringent safety protocols. Successful clinical trials hinge on meticulous planning and execution. Patient selection must prioritize individuals who are likely to benefit most while minimizing potential risks. This demands a clear understanding of the disease's genetic basis, the specific gene editing strategy, and the potential for adverse effects. Careful consideration of exclusion criteria is crucial to avoid enrolling participants who might experience complications. Furthermore, rigorous pre-clinical studies, using animal models and in vitro systems, are essential to establish efficacy and safety before human trials begin. These provide crucial data to support the safety and ethical conduct of human trials.

Effective monitoring of patient safety is paramount throughout all phases of clinical trials. This involves regular assessments of both intended and unintended consequences using a battery of techniques that vary based on the specific therapy. The frequency and intensity of monitoring should be tailored to the inherent risks associated with the gene editing procedure. These safety evaluations typically include comprehensive blood tests, imaging studies, and regular physical examinations to detect early signs of potential adverse events. Regularly scheduled safety review boards assess the ongoing safety and efficacy data to make decisions that protect the patients and provide oversight for the continued conduct of the clinical trial. These boards consist of independent experts who ensure the research adheres to ethical guidelines.

Securing regulatory approvals for gene editing therapies is a rigorous process requiring substantial documentation. This involves submitting comprehensive data packages to regulatory agencies, including pre-clinical and clinical trial results, demonstrating the therapy's safety and efficacy. Agencies, such as the FDA in the United States and the EMA in Europe, meticulously review this data using strict criteria. Compliance with Good Clinical Practice (GCP) guidelines, which dictate the ethical and scientific standards for clinical research, is essential. Demonstrating a clear understanding of the disease mechanism, the therapy's mechanism of action, and a thorough risk-benefit assessment are paramount for gaining approval. Failure to meet these stringent requirements can lead to delays or rejection of the application. The regulatory process often extends over several years, highlighting the complexities involved in introducing novel gene-editing therapies into clinical practice.

Patient safety protocols must be established and meticulously followed throughout the entire process, from initial screening to long-term follow-up. These protocols encompass a wide range of measures designed to mitigate potential risks. Informed consent is paramount, guaranteeing that patients fully understand the procedure, potential risks and benefits, and alternatives. Continuous monitoring of patients for adverse events is implemented using multiple methods that depend on the type of gene editing technique used and specific treatment administered. Post-treatment care plans, often complex and individualized, are critical to manage both immediate and potential long-term effects. Regular follow-up evaluations are crucial to assess both short-term and long-term efficacy and safety, as well as to detect and manage any delayed onset adverse effects.

Ultimately, the regulatory approval process and associated safety protocols are designed to balance the potential benefits of gene editing therapies with the inherent risks. While gene editing holds tremendous promise for treating a wide range of diseases, it's critical to proceed cautiously, implementing rigorous safety measures to protect patients. The success of gene editing technologies in clinical settings relies heavily on the responsible development of these therapies, adhering to ethical considerations, and complying with robust regulatory standards. The collaborative efforts of scientists, regulators, clinicians, and patients are indispensable in ensuring the safe and effective translation of gene editing from the laboratory to the clinic. This collaborative approach helps to ensure both the safety and efficacy of gene-editing therapies while also upholding the highest standards of ethical research practice.

7.1 Clinical Trial Design

Careful planning is paramount in gene therapy clinical trials. The initial phase, often a Phase I study, prioritizes safety. Researchers meticulously select a small group of participants, ensuring they meet specific inclusion criteria—for example, possessing the target genetic mutation and lacking other confounding health issues. This rigorous selection process minimizes risks and allows for close monitoring of any adverse events. Detailed protocols outline the dosage, administration method, and frequency of the gene therapy, as well as the procedures for monitoring participant health. Every step is meticulously documented, from participant recruitment to data analysis.

Data collection is extensive and systematic. Researchers monitor various biological parameters, conducting regular blood tests, imaging scans, and clinical assessments to gauge the treatment's effects. Genetic sequencing confirms the successful integration of the edited gene and monitors for off-target effects. This comprehensive data collection helps assess the safety and feasibility of the treatment, providing crucial information for subsequent trial phases. The data are analyzed frequently by statisticians to identify any emerging trends and to ensure the safety of participants.

Phase II trials expand the participant pool, allowing for a more thorough assessment of efficacy alongside safety. Researchers refine their approach based on learnings from Phase I. They might adjust dosages, delivery methods, or patient selection criteria to optimize the therapy's effectiveness while continuing to prioritize safety. A crucial component of Phase II is the assessment of biomarkers – biological indicators that correlate with treatment success or failure. This rigorous testing allows for a much deeper understanding of both treatment's effects and how it interacts with the human body.

Moving into Phase III, the clinical trial becomes a large-scale comparative study, usually against a placebo or the existing standard of care. Thousands of participants are recruited, enabling a strong statistical power to determine the treatment's true efficacy. This substantial sample size is critical for identifying rare adverse events and establishing the therapy's overall safety and effectiveness within a diverse population. Statistical analyses are crucial to assess if the gene editing treatment produces clinically meaningful improvements versus a control group. The meticulous nature of these late-stage clinical trials ensures unbiased and reliable results.

Beyond the core phases, post-market surveillance is crucial. Even after regulatory approval, continuous monitoring is vital. Researchers collect long-term data on participants to identify any late-onset effects, rare complications, or unexpected interactions with other medications. This ongoing process helps refine the therapy's usage guidelines, ensuring its safe and effective application in the long term. Continuous feedback from healthcare providers and patients is incorporated into this ongoing surveillance, enhancing the overall safety profile of the treatment. A robust system for reporting adverse events allows for swift action to address any concerns that may arise.

The design of a successful clinical trial necessitates a multidisciplinary team. Geneticists, clinicians, statisticians, and regulatory experts work in collaboration to ensure ethical conduct, scientific rigor, and efficient data management. Clear protocols, meticulously documented procedures, and robust data analysis systems are central to the success of each phase. Transparency and collaboration with regulatory bodies are key for navigating the complex approval process and ensuring the clinical trial's integrity. Each team member's expertise is indispensable in addressing various aspects of clinical trial design and execution.

Patient recruitment strategies are also critical. Trials must reach diverse populations to ensure the therapy's efficacy and safety are established across different demographics and genetic backgrounds. Outreach efforts include collaborations with patient advocacy groups, targeted advertising, and extensive screening protocols to identify suitable participants. Successful recruitment isn't simply about numbers but also about reaching the populations most likely to benefit and ensuring the diversity that creates a robust and meaningful data set. The process includes detailed informed consent procedures, meticulously explaining the risks and benefits of participation, and offering continuous support throughout the study. Clear communication with participants is critical.

7.2 Regulatory Approvals

Navigating the regulatory landscape for gene editing therapies can feel like traversing a complex maze. Success hinges on meticulous planning and a deep understanding of the multifaceted approval processes. Each step requires rigorous documentation, demonstrating not only efficacy but also the paramount importance of patient safety. This is not merely a bureaucratic hurdle; it's a crucial safeguard protecting patients and public trust in this rapidly evolving field.

The initial stages involve comprehensive pre-clinical studies, designed to rigorously test the safety and efficacy of the gene editing approach in vitro and in vivo. These studies must provide compelling evidence, demonstrating the therapy's ability to achieve the desired therapeutic effects while minimizing potential harm. Results must be meticulously documented and presented in a manner that clearly addresses potential concerns. Data supporting the safety profile–minimal off-target effects and avoidance of immune reactions–are especially vital at this stage. Consider the time investment; a thorough pre-clinical phase is essential for a strong application.

Next, you must meticulously plan your clinical trial design. This phase must follow stringent guidelines set by regulatory bodies such as the FDA in the United States or the EMA in Europe. Patient selection criteria are paramount; they must be precisely defined to ensure the inclusion of appropriate participants while excluding those who might be at higher risk. The selection process should be transparent and designed to avoid bias. Similarly, the trial protocol needs to detail every aspect of the trial, from the method of gene editing to the assessment of efficacy and safety endpoints. Detailed protocols aren't just paperwork, they form the foundation of any successful clinical trial.

Obtaining Investigational New Drug (IND) or Clinical Trial Application (CTA) approval represents a significant milestone. This requires the submission of a comprehensive application package, including all pre-clinical data, the clinical trial protocol, and information about the manufacturing process of the gene editing tools. Regulatory agencies scrutinize every detail, often requesting clarification or additional data. A strong application, supported by robust pre-clinical data and a well-defined clinical trial plan, will significantly increase the likelihood of approval. Transparency and comprehensive documentation are your allies in this critical phase.

Following the clinical trials, you must meticulously analyze the collected data. This involves not just assessing efficacy but also meticulously monitoring for adverse events and meticulously evaluating any safety concerns. Any unexpected findings must be promptly reported to the regulatory agency. The quality and rigor of data analysis directly influence the chances of securing approval. Think of this phase as your opportunity to provide conclusive evidence of both safety and efficacy.

The final stage, the New Drug Application (NDA) or Marketing Authorization Application (MAA), demands a comprehensive submission. This encompasses all data generated throughout the pre-clinical and clinical phases. Furthermore, it should include a thorough assessment of the manufacturing process, ensuring consistent quality and safety of the gene editing therapy. This stage also requires detailed plans for post-market surveillance, ensuring continued monitoring of the therapy's safety and efficacy once it enters the market. Careful preparation and comprehensive documentation are essential to navigate the final stage successfully. Don't underestimate the value of a well-prepared application.

Remember, effective communication with regulatory bodies is essential throughout the entire process. Proactive engagement, clear and concise documentation, and prompt responses to any requests or queries will help to streamline the process. This ongoing dialogue fosters a productive collaboration, ultimately helping in the safe and efficient introduction of life-changing gene editing therapies to patients. This collaborative approach is not just about approvals; it's about ensuring the responsible and ethical development of a revolutionary field.

7.3 Patient Safety Protocols

Rigorous screening of potential participants is paramount. Detailed medical histories, including family history of genetic disorders and any existing medical conditions, are meticulously reviewed. Extensive genetic testing is conducted to confirm the diagnosis and determine the specific genetic mutation, ensuring accurate targeting of the gene editing process. Only individuals with confirmed diagnoses and suitable genetic profiles proceed to further evaluation. This process minimizes risks associated with misdiagnosis or treating unsuitable candidates.

Pre-treatment evaluations extend beyond simple genetic screening. Comprehensive physical examinations, blood tests, imaging scans (where appropriate), and assessments of organ function are integral components of the screening process. This allows for a thorough understanding of the patient's overall health and baseline parameters, essential for monitoring treatment effects and identifying potential complications during and after the procedure. Identifying co-morbidities, though not necessarily exclusionary, requires careful risk-benefit assessment and specialized protocol adaptation.

The gene editing procedure itself necessitates a multidisciplinary approach. A team of specialists including geneticists, gene therapy experts, surgeons (if applicable), and anesthesiologists (if required), collaborate to ensure a safe and controlled environment for the procedure. Continuous monitoring of vital signs, oxygen saturation, and other physiological parameters are performed throughout the procedure by qualified medical professionals. This collaborative approach ensures the expertise of each medical discipline is leveraged for safety.

Post-procedure care involves comprehensive monitoring for any adverse effects or complications. Regular check-ups, including detailed physical examinations, blood tests, and genetic testing to assess the efficacy and safety of the gene editing process, are conducted. Follow-up appointments are scheduled at predetermined intervals, allowing for early detection and management of any complications. This includes close observation for signs of infection, inflammation, or immune responses.

Long-term follow-up is crucial for assessing the long-term safety and efficacy of the gene editing intervention. Regular follow-up visits, extending potentially over several years, allow for a thorough evaluation of sustained therapeutic benefits and the detection of any late-onset adverse effects. This long-term monitoring allows for the collection of critical data on the long-term consequences of the treatment and enables adjustments to future protocols based on these observations. Patient quality of life assessments are also integral to this process.

Data collected throughout the treatment process, from initial screening through long-term follow-up, is meticulously documented and analyzed. This data forms the basis for ongoing evaluation of the efficacy and safety of the protocols. Regular audits and reviews of these protocols, involving internal and potentially external experts, are necessary to identify areas for improvement and refinement. This systematic process allows for continuous refinement and enhancement of these protocols.

Strict adherence to good clinical practice (GCP) guidelines is non-negotiable. All aspects of the research, from study design to data analysis, must comply with international standards. Ethics committees play a vital role in the ongoing oversight of these protocols, providing continuous review and approval of the procedures ensuring ethical conduct and patient safety. These guidelines ensure adherence to the highest standards of safety and ethical conduct.

Comprehensive documentation of all procedures, including informed consent processes, treatment details, and post-treatment monitoring, are crucial. These records serve not only to pro vide detailed information about each patient's experience but also to contribute to the ongoing accumulation of knowledge and refinement of future safety protocols. Such detailed documentation is essential for transparency, accountability, and continuous improvement. This meticulous record-keeping enables rigorous analysis of treatment outcomes and facilitates identification of any adverse events.

Emergency preparedness and response plans must be in place to address potential complications. These plans detail the procedures to be followed in case of adverse events, ensuring timely and effective responses to any unforeseen circumstances. This includes clearly defined roles and responsibilities for medical personnel, ready access to emergency equipment and resources, and well-defined communication pathways. This proactive approach significantly enhances patient safety and reduces risks.

Open communication between healthcare providers and patients is crucial. Patients and their families must receive clear and concise information about the procedures, potential risks and benefits, and the importance of adherence to the post-treatment care plan. Regular opportunities for questions and discussion ensure that patients feel fully informed and empowered to participate actively in their own care. This open dialogue fosters a climate of trust and confidence.

www.ingramcontent.com/pod-product-compliance
Lightning Source LLC
LaVergne TN
LVHW022016200926
848481LV00007B/2418